CanMEDS 2015
Physician Competency Framework

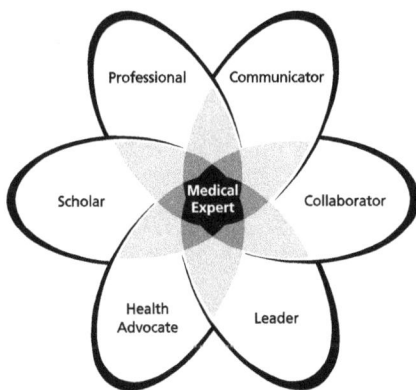

CANMEDS

EDITORS

Jason R. Frank

Linda Snell

Jonathan Sherbino

CanMEDS 2015 Physician Competency Framework

Royal College of Physicians and Surgeons of Canada
774 Echo Drive
Ottawa ON K1S 5N8
Canada

TOLL FREE 1 800-668-3740
TEL 613-730-8177
FAX 613-730-8262
WEB royalcollege.ca
EMAIL canmeds@royalcollege.ca

Printed in Canada.

ISBN: 978-1-926588-28-5

HOW TO CITE THIS DOCUMENT

Frank JR, Snell L, Sherbino J, editors. *CanMEDS 2015 Physician Competency Framework*. Ottawa: Royal College of Physicians and Surgeons of Canada; 2015.

HOW TO CITE INDIVIDUAL ROLES

Medical Expert

Bhanji F, Lawrence K, Goldszmidt M, Walton M, Harris K, Creery D, Sherbino J, Ste-Marie L-G, Stang A. Medical Expert. In: Frank JR, Snell L, Sherbino J, editors. *CanMEDS 2015 Physician Competency Framework*. Ottawa: Royal College of Physicians and Surgeons of Canada; 2015.

Communicator

Neville A, Weston W, Martin D, Samson L, Feldman P, Wallace G, Jamoulle O, François J, Lussier M-T, Dojeiji S. Communicator. In: Frank JR, Snell L, Sherbino J, editors. *CanMEDS 2015 Physician Competency Framework*. Ottawa: Royal College of Physicians and Surgeons of Canada; 2015.

Collaborator

Richardson D, Calder L, Dean H, Glover Takahashi S, Lebel P, Maniate J, Martin D, Nasmith L, Newton C, Steinert Y. Collaborator. In: Frank JR, Snell L, Sherbino J, editors. *CanMEDS 2015 Physician Competency Framework*. Ottawa: Royal College of Physicians and Surgeons of Canada; 2015.

Leader

Dath D, Chan M-K, Anderson G, Burke A, Razack S, Lieff S, Moineau G, Chiu A, Ellison P. Leader. In: Frank JR, Snell L, Sherbino J, editors. *CanMEDS 2015 Physician Competency Framework*. Ottawa: Royal College of Physicians and Surgeons of Canada; 2015.

Health Advocate

Sherbino J, Bonnycastle D, Côté B, Flynn L, Hunter A, Ince-Cushman D, Konkin J, Oandasan I, Regehr G, Richardson D, Zigby J. Health Advocate. In: Frank JR, Snell L, Sherbino J, editors. *CanMEDS 2015 Physician Competency Framework*. Ottawa: Royal College of Physicians and Surgeons of Canada; 2015.

Scholar

Richardson D, Oswald A, Chan M-K, Lang ES, Harvey BJ, editors. Scholar. In: Frank JR, Snell L, Sherbino J, editors. *CanMEDS 2015 Physician Competency Framework*. Ottawa: Royal College of Physicians and Surgeons of Canada; 2015.

Professional

Snell L, Flynn L, Pauls M, Kearney R, Warren A, Sternszus R, Cruess R, Cruess S, Hatala R, Dupré M, Bukowskyj M, Edwards S, Cohen J, Chakravarti A, Nickell L, Wright J. Professional. In: Frank JR, Snell L, Sherbino J, editors. *CanMEDS 2015 Physician Competency Framework*. Ottawa: Royal College of Physicians and Surgeons of Canada; 2015.

Contents

Foreword 4

Introduction

    The evolution of the CanMEDS Framework 5

    The CanMEDS 2015 project: objectives and principles 6

    The CanMEDS 2015 project and the Competence by Design initiative 7

    The CanMEDS 2015 project: a collaborative methodology 8

    Acknowledgments 9

Key features of the CanMEDS 2015 project: content changes by Role 10

Introducing milestones 12

Medical Expert 14

Communicator 16

Collaborator 18

Leader 20

Health Advocate 22

Scholar 24

Professional 26

A taxonomy of physician competencies 28

Key contributors 29

References 35

FOREWORD

The Fellows of the Royal College of Physicians and Surgeons of Canada (Royal College) are committed to improving the health and care of Canadians. The Royal College delivers on this mission in part by setting high standards for medical education and practice. These standards are informed by the CanMEDS Physician Competency Framework, which contributes directly to the delivery of quality health care.

Since its launch in 1996, CanMEDS has become the most widely accepted and widely applied physician competency framework in the world. Each revision that it undergoes is guided by extensive empirical research and wide consultation, and is based on evidence of societal need, Fellows' expertise and sound educational principles.

CanMEDS 2015 is the third edition of the framework and is in many ways our most significant revision. The Royal College began the CanMEDS renewal process as part of another multi-year initiative known as Competence by Design (CBD). CBD is an initiative to implement an enhanced model for competency-based medical education in residency training and specialty practice in Canada. Together the CanMEDS 2015 project and CBD resulted in rich new content within the CanMEDS Framework as well as new milestones to mark the progression of competence in each of the CanMEDS Roles across the continuum of medical education. The Milestones Guide, a companion resource, marks a major expansion of the CanMEDS vision and an important step toward integrating competency based curricula in postgraduate programs, as was recommended in 2012 by The Future of Medical Education in Canada Postgraduate Project, a Canadian collaborative initiative.[1]

The development of this 2015 edition of the framework was a truly collaborative effort. It saw the participation of hundreds of dedicated medical educators, clinicians, learners, committee members, and staff. Moreover, numerous organizations involved in medical education in Canada and around the world also contributed their expertise, and we are proud to say that many of Canada's leading medical education organizations formally endorse the CanMEDS 2015 Framework.

It is with great pleasure that we present the CanMEDS 2015 Physician Competency Framework. We trust that it will be useful to all those who care about physician competence and quality health care.

Kevin Imrie,
MD, FRCPC, FACP
President

Andrew Padmos,
BA, MD, FRCPC, FACP
Chief Executive Officer

Kenneth A. Harris,
MD, FRCSC
Executive Director,
Office of Specialty Education
and Deputy CEO

The evolution of the CanMEDS Framework

How much has happened in these 50 years — a period more remarkable than any, I will continue to say...I am thinking of those revolutions in science which have...changed the position and prospects of [humankind]...[2]
— Benjamin Disraeli, 1873

Medical education is changing rapidly, and CanMEDS is part of that story. CanMEDS is, at its heart, an initiative to improve patient care by enhancing physician training. From the beginning, its main purpose has been to articulate a comprehensive definition of the abilities needed for all domains of medical practice and thus provide a strong foundation for medical education.

In the early 1990s, Fellows of the Royal College of Physicians and Surgeons of Canada, with support from the charitable institution Associated Medical Services, leveraged the important work of the Educating Future Physicians for Ontario project to develop a competency framework for specialist physicians.[3, 4] The result, the CanMEDS Framework, was formally approved by the Royal College in 1996 and subsequently updated in 2005.[5, 6] CanMEDS is now used in dozens of countries on five continents, in medicine and in other health care professions, making it the most recognized and most widely applied health care profession competency framework in the world. The Royal College continues to be the steward and sponsor of the framework, and the current iteration was prepared with input from major medical institutions around the world.

In Canada, CanMEDS forms the basis for all Royal College educational standards for specialty education. The College of Family Physicians of Canada has in recent years formally integrated an adaptation known as CanMEDS-FM (CanMEDS–Family Medicine) into the training of all family physicians in Canada. CanMEDS has also been adopted by the Collège des médecins du Québec, the Medical Council of Canada, the Canadian Medical Association and Canada's medical schools. The use of a national competency-based framework for medical training is one reason why the Canadian medical education system is regarded as among the strongest in the world.

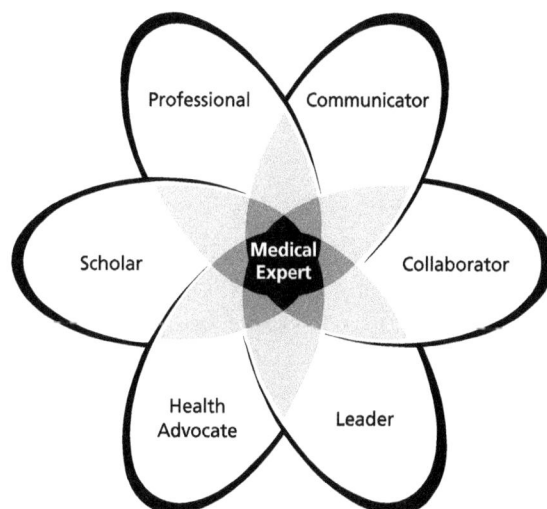

CanMEDS

INTRODUCTION

The CanMEDS 2015 project: objectives and principles

To help prepare physicians meet societal needs in a dynamic and increasingly demanding health care environment, those stewarding CanMEDS remain committed to keeping the framework current and to facilitating its implementation in the real world of medical education and practice.

The CanMEDS 2015 project set out to meet the following objectives, while working within the existing CanMEDS Roles:

1. Add new themes emerging in health care, such as patient safety, eHealth and handover.

2. Address the needs of front-line educators who had asked for practical changes and updates that make it easier to teach and assess the CanMEDS Roles.

3. Develop new competency milestones that support the practical application of the framework in residency training programs and throughout a physician's career.

To meet these objectives, the participants in the CanMEDS 2015 revision process adopted the following guidelines as foundational to their work:

- The process is one of revision and renewal: improvement, not reinvention, is the goal.

- The primary target audiences comprise trainees, front-line teachers, program directors of various curricula and clinician educators who design programs.

- The competency constructs need to be grounded in theory and best practices, while their presentation needs to be realistic and related to the daily practice of any physician.

- Competencies are to be articulated in a generic manner to facilitate their adaptation by all specialties.

- Concepts that are relevant to multiple Roles will be articulated in the Role where they are the most prominent. Although redundancy and overlap are accepted, and even expected, the framework itself will avoid repetition while ensuring the appropriate integration of Roles.

"With the many changes occurring in the medical workforce, there is a pressing need to make sure that CanMEDS 2015 reflects the values of the next generation of physicians."

Source: CanMEDS 2015 Consultations. Written submission.

The CanMEDS 2015 project and the Competence by Design initiative

The CanMEDS 2015 project is foundational to another key initiative of the Royal College known as Competence by Design.[7] Competence by Design is a multi-year project to implement an enhanced model for competency-based medical education (CBME) in residency training and specialty practice in Canada. Both CanMEDS and Competence by Design are part of a worldwide trend toward CBME now under way.

The aim of the Competence by Design project is to transform Canadian medical training. The move to competency-based medical education is seen as a mechanism to enhance the practice readiness of graduates and ensure they leave supervised training with the skills needed to continue their learning throughout their professional career. This requires a move away from traditional time-based immersions with an emphasis on a single point in time assessment to a system of demonstrating performance regularly in real situations and settings. Through the CanMEDS 2015 Framework, and the associated CanMEDS milestones, educators now have useful markers of progression to use as the basis for meaningful feedback to learners. Learners will use this feedback to both enhance and record their educational progress.

The Royal College's Competence by Design project is ready to provide leadership for medical education worldwide. Working in collaboration with a consortium of key partners in Canada, we are bringing the implementation of CBME within reach. Competence by Design will influence the delivery of medical education in Canada and beyond.

COMPETENCY-BASED MEDICAL EDUCATION: KEY DEFINITIONS[8]

Competency-based medical education (CBME): An approach to designing medical training that is focused on outcomes in the form of the abilities of graduates

Competency: An observable ability of a health care professional that develops through stages of expertise from novice to master clinician

Entrustable professional activity (EPA): A key task of a discipline that can be entrusted to an individual who possesses the appropriate level of competence

Milestone: The expected ability of a health care professional at a stage of expertise

"The movement to identify competencies over the physician's practice lifetime is an important CanMEDS evolution, enabling the application of the framework beyond residency [and the] entry to practice."

Source: CanMEDS 2015 Consultations. Written submission.

INTRODUCTION

The CanMEDS 2015 project: a collaborative methodology

Those who use the CanMEDS Framework in education and practice need to be confident that it is a valid and practical foundation for excellence in patient care. Since its beginning in the 1990s, CanMEDS has been the product of an evidence-informed, collaborative process involving hundreds, if not thousands, of Royal College Fellows, family physicians, educators, learners and other expert volunteers.

Its development has involved countless hours of literature reviews, stakeholder surveys, focus groups, interviews, consultations, consensus-building exercises, debate and work on educational design. Many people in Canada and around the world feel that the strength of the CanMEDS Framework lies in the fact that it was derived explicitly from societal needs.

For the CanMEDS 2015 project, the Royal College engaged as diverse a cadre of experts and partners as possible to ensure that the new version of the framework was comprehensive and practical. In early 2013, the Royal College commissioned a series of committees and 13 Expert Working Groups (EWGs), which then set out to revise aspects of CanMEDS. Participants were recruited for a range of reasons, including their subject matter expertise, their perspective on a particular stage of physician development (e.g. learning in practice), their understanding of the health care and medical education systems, and their geography. A list of committee and EWG members is found at the end of this document.

To engage the profession, we chose an elaborate global consensus process as our methodology. Each EWG was tasked with reviewing the recent literature and reports relevant to a subdomain of CanMEDS and reporting back their recommendations for new standards. All of these working group reports can be found on the web.[9] As was done for the original 1996 framework, we conducted focus groups and surveys with health care professionals and members of the public to get a variety of perspectives on the abilities people expect and need from their physicians.[10] A National and an International Advisory Committee each gave iterative feedback as

reports came in. An overarching Integration Committee performed the Herculean task of editing the vast data into successive versions of a coherent new framework. Finally, a dedicated group of bilingual physicians chaired by Dr. Andrée Boucher wrote a version of the framework and milestones *en français*.[11]

The CanMEDS 2015 Framework was developed in collaboration with 12 medical education organizations as part of their work on the CanMEDS 2015 National Advisory Committee. Each of the Association of Faculties of Medicine of Canada, the Canadian Federation of Medical Students, the Canadian Medical Association, the Canadian Medical Protective Association, the Canadian Patient Safety Institute, the Collège des médecins du Québec, the College of Family Physicians of Canada, the Fédération des médecins résidents du Québec, the Fédération médicale étudiante du Québec, the Federation of Medical Regulatory Authorities of Canada, the Medical Council of Canada and the Resident Doctors of Canada has endorsed the use of the CanMEDS 2015 Physician Competency Framework to inform each organization's work, adapting it for their own specific context.

Key Contributors to the CanMEDS 2015 Project:

- CanMEDS 2015 National Advisory Committee
- CanMEDS 2015 Integration Committee
- 13 CanMEDS 2015 Expert Working Groups
- CanMEDS 2015 International Advisory Committee
- Royal College French Advisory Committee

Acknowledgments

This update to the Royal College CanMEDS Physician Competency Framework as well as the development of competency milestones could not have been accomplished without the participation of hundreds of dedicated medical educators, clinicians, residents, medical students, committee members, and staff.

This effort was about revision and renewal, not reinvention, and we therefore also gratefully acknowledge the work of the contributors to the 1996 and 2005 editions.

We greatly appreciate the dedicated work of the many members of the Expert Working Groups, the Integration Committee, the National Advisory Committee and the International Advisory Committee, all of whom are listed at the end of this document.

The commitment and expertise of the chairs of the Expert Working Groups deserve special mention. Thank you to Farhan Bhanji, Andrée Boucher, Ming-Ka Chan, Deepak Dath, Leslie Flynn, Bart Harvey, Kendall Ho, Eddy Lang, Alan Neville, Anna Oswald, Denyse Richardson, Jonathan Sherbino, Linda Snell and Brian Wong. Sincere thanks also to Elaine Van Melle for her scholarly and research support to the Expert Working Groups and Royal College staff throughout the project.

We also recognize the important work of the CanMEDS 2015 Project Secretariat. We thank the team for its contribution to this truly collaborative and consultative review process.

Finally, we thank all of the other participants in the CanMEDS 2015 project: the Royal College French Advisory Committee, ePanelists, focus group participants, survey respondents and the hundreds of participants in town hall meetings. Their input helped ensure the utility and validity of the CanMEDS 2015 Framework and the associated CanMEDS Milestones Guide.

Jason R Frank MD MA(Ed) FRCPC
Editor, CanMEDS 2015 Framework and CanMEDS Milestones Guide
Co-chair, National & International Advisory Committees

Linda Snell MD MHPE FRCPC MACP
Editor, CanMEDS 2015 Framework and CanMEDS Milestones Guide
Co-chair, International Advisory Committee

Jonathan Sherbino MD MEd FRCPC
Editor, CanMEDS 2015 Framework and CanMEDS Milestones Guide

Ivy F Oandasan MD CCFP MHSc FCFP
Co-chair, National Advisory Committee

Cynthia Abbott MPl
Manager, CanMEDS and Faculty Development

KEY CHANGES

Key features of the CanMEDS 2015 project: content changes by Role

The following summaries highlight general changes and changes by Role as a result of the CanMEDS 2015 project.

General changes

- There is a renewed emphasis on the overall coherence of the framework, and on accessible language that supports practical application.

- Role descriptions and definitions are expressed in simpler, more direct language.

- Areas of overlap between Roles are minimized, resulting in a 3.5% decrease in the number of key competencies and a 29.4% decrease in the number of enabling competencies; although aspects of a shared plan of care may pertain to more than one Role, the competencies of a given Role are written specifically for that Role alone.

- The addition of complementary milestones provides clearly defined targets to guide learning and assessment and mark the progression of competence throughout a physician's career.

- Competencies and milestones describe the abilities to be demonstrated in practice, as distinct from the information or content related to aspects of a Role.

- Competencies related to safeguarding and enhancing patient safety are integrated throughout the framework and milestones, as recommended by the Patient Safety and Quality Improvement EWG and validated in early consultations.

- Competencies associated with eHealth are integrated throughout the framework and milestones, as recommended by the eHealth EWG and validated in consultations.

- There is a new online glossary of key terms associated with the framework.

- A new CanMEDS diagram reflects the quality improvements achieved in the 2015 revisions.

Medical Expert

- The definition, description and first key competency of the Medical Expert Role highlight the importance of integrating the six Intrinsic Roles.[12]

- The concepts of complexity, uncertainty and ambiguity are now more explicit.

- The Role reflects some of the complexity in decision-making and clinical reasoning that occurs before, during and after the completion of procedures.

- A key competency addresses the evolving recognition of patient safety and continuous quality improvement as important components of medical expertise at the bedside.

Communicator

- The scope of the Communicator Role now focuses exclusively on the interaction between physicians and their patients, including patients' families.*

- Patient-centred and therapeutic communication is emphasized.

- Communication with other colleagues in the health care professions is now covered explicitly in the Collaborator Role.

- The concept of cultural safety is now explicit.

---

* Throughout the CanMEDS 2015 Framework and Milestones Guide, references to the patient's family are intended to include all those who are personally significant to the patient and are concerned with his or her care, including, according to the patient's circumstances, family members, partners, caregivers, legal guardians, and substitute decision-makers.

Collaborator

- A new key competency addresses handovers and care transitions.
- The concept of collaboration among physicians is given explicit emphasis.
- A relationship-centred model of care is used to organize these competencies.
- Value is placed on including the patient's perspective in the shared decision-making process.
- Collaboration is reflected more broadly, to extend beyond the context of a formalized health care team.

Leader

- A name change for the Role from "Manager" to "Leader" reflects an emphasis on the leadership skills needed by physicians to contribute to the ongoing improvement of health care.
- Competence in patient safety and quality improvement has a new emphasis, including contributing to a culture that promotes patient safety.
- Emphasis is placed on the development of skills to achieve balance between professional practice and personal life.
- Resource allocation is conceived as a function of good stewardship.
- Competence in health informatics is viewed as crucial for medical leaders and managers and as vital to the delivery of health care.

Health Advocate

- Now includes an expanded and refined definition and description.
- Includes the notion of partnership in advocacy.

Scholar

- The "lifelong learner" component of the Scholar Role is organized into three enabling competencies that reflect (1) the need for a personal learning plan, (2) the use of data from a variety of sources to guide learning, and (3) the importance of collaborative learning.

- The concepts of patient safety and a safe learning environment are explicit in the "teacher" component of the Role.
- A new key competency on evidence-informed practice is included.
- There is a new emphasis on skills in structured critical appraisal.
- The concept of research is broader, emphasizing that physicians not only participate in research but also are involved in the dissemination of research findings.

Professional

- Key competencies are organized to reflect the commitment of the physician to the patient, to society and to the profession.
- There is now an increased emphasis on physician health and well-being.
- The emerging concept of professional identity formation is woven throughout the Professional Role.[13]

"We urge you to try and organize issues in one category only, to avoid duplication and repetition — this will assist with applying this framework, e.g. tracking data, creating templates, providing feedback, creating practice improvement plans, and [facilitating] Continuing Professional Development."
Source: CanMEDS 2015 Consultations. Written submission.

"There are a number of themes that should be expressed across all Roles... we particularly support the decision to include patient safety..."
Source: CanMEDS 2015 Consultations. Written submission.

MILESTONES

Introducing milestones

Unlike previous editions, CanMEDS 2015 is part of a larger project: Competence by Design (CBD). CBD is a move away from credentialing physicians solely on the basis of time spent on rotations and activities in favour of ensuring achievement on the basis of attained milestones of competence.

The addition of complementary milestones is arguably the biggest change between the 2005 and the 2015 versions of the CanMEDS Framework. The milestones are presented separately in the CanMEDS Milestones Guide, a companion document that can be found online. Unlike the CanMEDS Framework, which will change infrequently, the Milestones will undergo continual revision as educators modify them for their discipline. The Milestones Guide provides opportunity for dialogue among educators working across the continuum of learning (i.e., undergraduate, postgraduate, continuing professional development). Descriptions used in the Milestones Guide can help educators enhance the learners' transition from one stage of learning to the next.

The 2005 Framework describes the competencies expected of trainees at the end of their formal education (i.e., at the point when they are "ready" to enter practice). Although all trainees and their program directors know from the start what competencies are expected of them by the end of their training, until now no standard expectations have been articulated for other phases of their career. The milestones introduce descriptions of the abilities expected of a trainee or physician at defined stages of professional development.

"We believe that in the future, expertise rather than experience will underlie competency-based practice and ... certification."[14]
(Aggarwal & Darzi 2006)

The Royal College uses milestones to:

- mark the progression of competence throughout a physician's career;

- provide clearly defined targets to guide learning and assessment — targets that are based in real-life, meaningful learning experiences;

- enable learners to focus their learning activities more effectively; and

- enable assessors (and programs) to know when a learner has achieved a given milestone or set of milestones and is truly ready to move to the next stage of training or development.

The CanMEDS 2015 Milestones are a guide to help medical educators describe the progression of competence for each discipline. We do not expect that educators will use all of the milestones when tailoring the CanMEDS Framework to their discipline or educational context.

MILESTONES AND THE COMPETENCY-BASED APPROACH

By introducing a next-generation competency-based medical education (CBME) model into trainee learning and specialty practice, the CBD initiative breaks down specialist education into a series of integrated stages, starting with the transition to discipline and moving through practice. (See diagram on p. 13).

Each stage incorporates milestones that define the specific abilities expected at certain points within a physician's career. By focusing on learning rather than time, the CBD approach is helping the Royal College align medical education with the realities of today's practice and thus ensure that physicians have the competencies they need at every stage of their career.

MEDICAL EDUCATION PHASES AND STAGES

Physicians develop competencies at different stages during discipline-specific residency and throughout practice.

Discipline-specific residency. This phase is the period in which a physician trainee builds upon the foundational abilities acquired in medical school to learn the competencies needed for practice. It comprises four advancing stages: transition to discipline, foundations of discipline, core of discipline, and transition to practice.

- **Transition to discipline.** In many cases this is a new addition to the residency phase of medical education. This stage emphasizes the orientation and assessment of new trainees arriving from different medical schools and programs (including outside Canada). Although this stage does exist in some form in many residency programs (e.g. residency "boot camps"), the CBD approach formalizes the assessment and orientation process, ensuring a level playing field for residents as they begin their specialist training. This stage may require a day, a month, or two months, depending on the needs of each program and of individual learners.

- **Foundations of discipline.** The second stage in the residency phase covers broad-based competencies that every trainee must acquire before moving on to more advanced discipline-specific competencies. This may involve rotating through a number of clinical settings so the trainee can acquire a breadth of foundational abilities to prepare for core training.

- **Core of discipline.** The third stage in the residency phase covers the core competencies that make up the majority of a discipline.*

- **Transition to practice.** In the final stage in the residency phase of medical education, the senior trainee should demonstrate readiness to make the transition to autonomous practice: for example, acting as a chief resident, running an ambulatory clinic, performing procedures with increasing autonomy, and teaching others. Royal College certification will be granted upon the successful completion of the "transition to practice" stage.

Continuing professional development (CPD). A physician maintains and enhances competence throughout practice in the following ways:

- **Maintenance of competence.** A physician engages in CPD to remain up-to-date and sustain expertise within his or her scope of practice.

- **Advanced expertise.** The physician acquires new or expanded skills and abilities so that his or her practice can evolve over time in response to practice needs and interests.

- **Transition out of professional practice.** In this last stage, physicians adapt to the final practice period and their changing health care role.

CBD[1,2] Competence Continuum

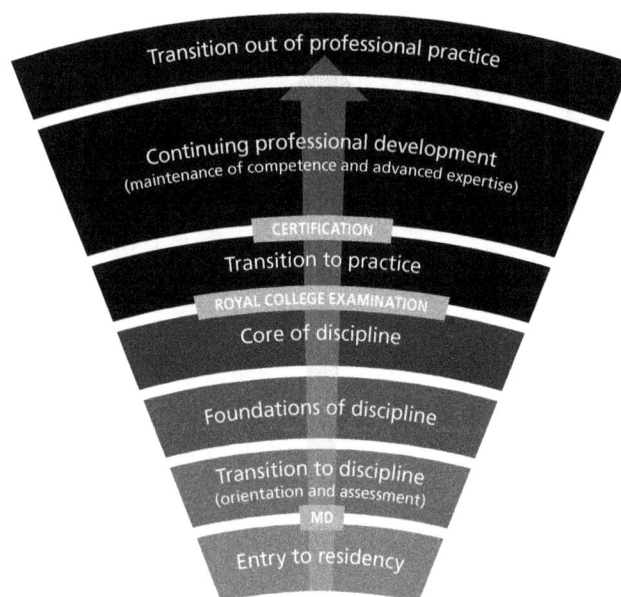

[1] Competence by Design (CBD)
[2] Milestones at each stage describe terminal competencies

---

* Royal College examination: The CBD approach proposes that the Royal College examination be taken at the end of the "core of discipline" stage, rather than at the end of the training stage, where it currently sits. Moving the exam will ensure trainees are able to focus on further clinical training in their final year, allowing them to use their final supervised training time to hone competencies. Emphasis could then be placed on increasingly independent work and skills — creating physicians who are truly ready for independent practice.

Medical Expert

MEDICAL EXPERT

DEFINITION

As Medical Experts, physicians integrate all of the CanMEDS Roles, applying medical knowledge, clinical skills, and professional values in their provision of high-quality and safe patient-centred care. Medical Expert is the central physician Role in the CanMEDS Framework and defines the physician's clinical scope of practice.

DESCRIPTION

As Medical Experts who provide high-quality, safe, patient-centred care, physicians draw upon an evolving body of knowledge, their clinical skills, and their professional values. They collect and interpret information, make clinical decisions, and carry out diagnostic and therapeutic interventions. They do so within their scope of practice and with an understanding of the limits of their expertise. Their decision-making is informed by best practices and research evidence, and takes into account the patient's circumstances and preferences as well as the availability of resources. Their clinical practice is up-to-date, ethical, and resource-efficient, and is conducted in collaboration with patients and their families,* other health care professionals, and the community. The Medical Expert Role is central to the function of physicians and draws on the competencies included in the Intrinsic Roles (Communicator, Collaborator, Leader, Health Advocate, Scholar, and Professional).

KEY CONCEPTS

Agreed-upon goals of care: 2.1, 2.3, 2.4, 3.2, 4.1

Application of core clinical and biomedical sciences: 1.3

Clinical decision-making: 1.4, 1.6, 2.2

Clinical reasoning: 1.3, 1.4, 2.1, 3.1

Compassion: 1.1

Complexity, uncertainty, and ambiguity in clinical decision-making: 1.6, 2.2, 2.4, 3.2, 3.3, 3.4

Consent: 3.2

Continuity of care: 2.4, 4.1

Duty of care: 1.1, 1.5, 2.4

Integration of CanMEDS Intrinsic Roles: 1.2

Interpreting diagnostic tests: 2.2

Medical expertise: all enabling competencies

Patient-centred clinical assessment and management: 1.4, 2.2, 2.4, 3.1, 3.3, 3.4, 4.1, 5.2

Patient safety: 1.5, 3.4, 5.1, 5.2

Prioritization of professional responsibilities: 1.4, 1.5, 2.1, 3.3, 5.1

Procedural skill proficiency: 3.1, 3.3, 3.4

Quality improvement: 5.1, 5.2

Self-awareness of limits of expertise: 1.4, 3.4

Timely follow-up: 1.4, 2.2, 4.1

Working within the health care team: 1.3, 1.4, 2.1, 2.4, 3.3, 4.1, 5.1

---

* Throughout the CanMEDS 2015 Framework and Milestones Guide, references to the patient's family are intended to include all those who are personally significant to the patient and are concerned with his or her care, including, according to the patient's circumstances, family members, partners, caregivers, legal guardians, and substitute decision-makers.

MEDICAL EXPERT

Key competencies	Enabling competencies
PHYSICIANS ARE ABLE TO:	
1. **Practise medicine within their defined scope of practice and expertise**	1.1 Demonstrate a commitment to high-quality care of their patients
	1.2 Integrate the CanMEDS Intrinsic Roles into their practice of medicine
	1.3 Apply knowledge of the clinical and biomedical sciences relevant to their discipline
	1.4 Perform appropriately timed clinical assessments with recommendations that are presented in an organized manner
	1.5 Carry out professional duties in the face of multiple, competing demands
	1.6 Recognize and respond to the complexity, uncertainty, and ambiguity inherent in medical practice
2. **Perform a patient-centred clinical assessment and establish a management plan**	2.1 Prioritize issues to be addressed in a patient encounter
	2.2 Elicit a history, perform a physical exam, select appropriate investigations, and interpret their results for the purpose of diagnosis and management, disease prevention, and health promotion
	2.3 Establish goals of care in collaboration with patients and their families, which may include slowing disease progression, treating symptoms, achieving cure, improving function, and palliation
	2.4 Establish a patient-centred management plan
3. **Plan and perform procedures and therapies for the purpose of assessment and/or management**	3.1 Determine the most appropriate procedures or therapies
	3.2 Obtain and document informed consent, explaining the risks and benefits of, and the rationale for, a proposed procedure or therapy
	3.3 Prioritize a procedure or therapy, taking into account clinical urgency and available resources
	3.4 Perform a procedure in a skilful and safe manner, adapting to unanticipated findings or changing clinical circumstances
4. **Establish plans for ongoing care and, when appropriate, timely consultation**	4.1 Implement a patient-centred care plan that supports ongoing care, follow-up on investigations, response to treatment, and further consultation
5. **Actively contribute, as an individual and as a member of a team providing care, to the continuous improvement of health care quality and patient safety**	5.1 Recognize and respond to harm from health care delivery, including patient safety incidents
	5.2 Adopt strategies that promote patient safety and address human and system factors

Communicator

DEFINITION

As Communicators, physicians form relationships with patients and their families* that facilitate the gathering and sharing of essential information for effective health care.†

DESCRIPTION

Physicians enable patient-centred therapeutic communication by exploring the patient's symptoms, which may be suggestive of disease, and by actively listening to the patient's experience of his or her illness. Physicians explore the patient's perspective, including his or her fears, ideas about the illness, feelings about the impact of the illness, and expectations of health care and health care professionals. The physician integrates this knowledge with an understanding of the patient's context, including socio-economic status, medical history, family history, stage of life, living situation, work or school setting, and other relevant psychological and social issues. Central to a patient-centred approach is shared decision-making: finding common ground with the patient in developing a plan to address his or her medical problems and health goals in a manner that reflects the patient's needs, values, and preferences. This plan should be informed by evidence and guidelines.

Because illness affects not only patients but also their families, physicians must be able to communicate effectively with everyone involved in the patient's care.

KEY CONCEPTS

Accuracy: 2.1, 3.1, 4.2, 5.1

Active listening: 1.1, 1.3, 1.4, 1.5, 2.1, 2.2, 2.3, 4.1, 4.3

Appropriate documentation: 2.1, 5.1, 5.2, 5.3

Attention to the psychosocial aspects of illness: 1.6, 2.1, 2.2, 4.1

Breaking bad news: 1.5, 3.1

Concordance of goals and expectations: 1.6, 2.2, 3.1, 4.3

Disclosure of harmful patient safety incidents: 3.2

Effective oral and written information for patient care across different media: 5.1, 5.2, 5.3

Efficiency: 2.3, 4.2, 5.2

Eliciting and synthesizing information for patient care: 2.1, 2.2, 2.3

Empathy: 1.1, 1.2, 1.3

Ethics in the physician–patient encounter: 3.2, 5.1

Expert verbal and non-verbal communication: 1.1, 1.4

Informed consent: 2.2

Mutual understanding: 1.6, 3.1, 4.1

Patient-centred approach to communication: 1.1, 1.6, 2.1, 3.1

Privacy and confidentiality: 1.2, 5.1

Rapport: 1.4

Relational competence in interactions: 1.5

Respect for diversity: 1.1, 1.6, 2.2, 4.1

Shared decision-making: 1.6, 4.1, 4.3

Therapeutic relationships with patients and their families: 1.2, 1.3, 1.4, 1.5, 1.6

Transition in care: 5.1, 5.2, 5.3

Trust in the physician–patient relationship: 1.1, 5.2, 5.3

---

* Throughout the CanMEDS 2015 Framework and Milestones Guide, references to the patient's family are intended to include all those who are personally significant to the patient and are concerned with his or her care, including, according to the patient's circumstances, family members, partners, caregivers, legal guardian, and substitute decision-makers.

† Note that the Communicator Role describes the abilities related to a physician–patient encounter. Other communication skills are found elsewhere in the framework, including health care team communication (Collaborator) and academic presentations (Scholar).

COMMUNICATOR

Key competencies	Enabling competencies
PHYSICIANS ARE ABLE TO:	
1. **Establish professional therapeutic relationships with patients and their families**	1.1 Communicate using a patient-centred approach that encourages patient trust and autonomy and is characterized by empathy, respect, and compassion
	1.2 Optimize the physical environment for patient comfort, dignity, privacy, engagement, and safety
	1.3 Recognize when the values, biases, or perspectives of patients, physicians, or other health care professionals may have an impact on the quality of care, and modify the approach to the patient accordingly
	1.4 Respond to a patient's non-verbal behaviours to enhance communication
	1.5 Manage disagreements and emotionally charged conversations
	1.6 Adapt to the unique needs and preferences of each patient and to his or her clinical condition and circumstances
2. **Elicit and synthesize accurate and relevant information, incorporating the perspectives of patients and their families**	2.1 Use patient-centred interviewing skills to effectively gather relevant biomedical and psychosocial information
	2.2 Provide a clear structure for and manage the flow of an entire patient encounter
	2.3 Seek and synthesize relevant information from other sources, including the patient's family, with the patient's consent
3. **Share health care information and plans with patients and their families**	3.1 Share information and explanations that are clear, accurate, and timely, while checking for patient and family understanding
	3.2 Disclose harmful patient safety incidents to patients and their families accurately and appropriately
4. **Engage patients and their families in developing plans that reflect the patient's health care needs and goals**	4.1 Facilitate discussions with patients and their families in a way that is respectful, non-judgmental, and culturally safe
	4.2 Assist patients and their families to identify, access, and make use of information and communication technologies to support their care and manage their health
	4.3 Use communication skills and strategies that help patients and their families make informed decisions regarding their health
5. **Document and share written and electronic information about the medical encounter to optimize clinical decision-making, patient safety, confidentiality, and privacy**	5.1 Document clinical encounters in an accurate, complete, timely, and accessible manner, in compliance with regulatory and legal requirements
	5.2 Communicate effectively using a written health record, electronic medical record, or other digital technology
	5.3 Share information with patients and others in a manner that respects patient privacy and confidentiality and enhances understanding

Collaborator

COLLABORATOR

DEFINITION

As Collaborators, physicians work effectively with other health care professionals to provide safe, high-quality, patient-centred care.

DESCRIPTION

Collaboration is essential for safe, high-quality, patient-centred care, and involves patients and their families,* physicians and other colleagues in the health care professions, community partners, and health system stakeholders.

Collaboration requires relationships based in trust, respect, and shared decision-making among a variety of individuals with complementary skills in multiple settings across the continuum of care. It involves sharing knowledge, perspectives, and responsibilities, and a willingness to learn together. This requires understanding the roles of others, pursuing common goals and outcomes, and managing differences.

Collaboration skills are broadly applicable to activities beyond clinical care, such as administration, education, advocacy, and scholarship.

KEY CONCEPTS

Collaboration with community providers: 1.1, 1.2, 1.3

Communities of practice: 1.3, 3.2

Conflict resolution, management, and prevention: 2.2

Constructive negotiation: 2.2

Effective consultation and referral: 1.2, 1.3, 3.1, 3.2

Effective health care teams: all enabling competencies

Handover: 3.1, 3.2

Interprofessional (i.e. among health care professionals) health care: all enabling competencies

Intraprofessional (i.e. among physician colleagues) health care: all enabling competencies

Recognizing one's own roles and limits: 1.2, 3.1

Relationship-centred care: all enabling competencies

Respect for other physicians and members of the health care team: 2.1, 2.2

Respecting and valuing diversity: 1.2, 2.1, 2.2

Shared decision-making: 1.3

Sharing of knowledge and information: 1.3, 3.1, 3.2

Situational awareness: 1.1, 1.2, 2.2, 3.1, 3.2

Team dynamics: 1.1, 2.2, 3.1

Transitions of care: 3.1, 3.2

---

* Throughout the CanMEDS 2015 Framework and Milestones Guide, references to the patient's family are intended to include all those who are personally significant to the patient and are concerned with his or her care, including, according to the patient's circumstances, family members, partners, caregivers, legal guardians, and substitute decision-makers.

COLLABORATOR

Key competencies	Enabling competencies
PHYSICIANS ARE ABLE TO:	
1. **Work effectively with physicians and other colleagues in the health care professions**	1.1 Establish and maintain positive relationships with physicians and other colleagues in the health care professions to support relationship-centred collaborative care
	1.2 Negotiate overlapping and shared responsibilities with physicians and other colleagues in the health care professions in episodic and ongoing care
	1.3 Engage in respectful shared decision-making with physicians and other colleagues in the health care professions
2. **Work with physicians and other colleagues in the health care professions to promote understanding, manage differences, and resolve conflicts**	2.1 Show respect toward collaborators
	2.2 Implement strategies to promote understanding, manage differences, and resolve conflicts in a manner that supports a collaborative culture
3. **Hand over the care of a patient to another health care professional to facilitate continuity of safe patient care**	3.1 Determine when care should be transferred to another physician or health care professional
	3.2 Demonstrate safe handover of care, using both verbal and written communication, during a patient transition to a different health care professional, setting, or stage of care

LEADER

Leader

DEFINITION

As Leaders, physicians engage with others to contribute to a vision of a high-quality health care system and take responsibility for the delivery of excellent patient care through their activities as clinicians, administrators, scholars, or teachers.

DESCRIPTION

The CanMEDS Leader Role describes the engagement of all physicians in shared decision-making for the operation and ongoing evolution of the health care system. As a societal expectation, physicians demonstrate collaborative leadership and management within the health care system. At a system level, physicians contribute to the development and delivery of continuously improving health care and engage with others in working toward this goal. Physicians integrate their personal lives with their clinical, administrative, scholarly, and teaching responsibilities. They function as individual care providers, as members of teams, and as participants and leaders in the health care system locally, regionally, nationally, and globally.

KEY CONCEPTS

Administration: 4.1, 4.2

Career development: 4.2

Complexity of systems: 1.1

Consideration of justice, efficiency, and effectiveness in the allocation of health care resources: 1.1, 1.2, 1.3, 1.4, 2.1, 2.2

Effective committee participation: 3.2

Health human resources: 2.1, 4.2

Information technology for health care: 1.4

Leading change: 1.1, 1.2, 1.3, 1.4, 2.2, 3.2

Management of personnel: 4.2

Negotiation: 3.1

Organizing, structuring, budgeting, and financing: 2.1, 2.2, 4.1, 4.2, 4.3

Personal leadership skills: 3.1, 4.1

Physician remuneration: 4.2

Physician roles and responsibilities in the health care system: 1.1, 1.2, 1.3, 1.4, 2.2, 3.2

Physicians as active participant-architects within the health care system: 1.1, 1.2, 1.3, 1.4, 3.2

Practice management to maintain a sustainable practice and physician health: 4.1, 4.2, 4.3

Priority-setting: 2.1, 3.2, 4.1

Quality improvement: 1.1, 1.2, 1.3, 1.4, 2.2, 3.2, 4.3

Stewardship: 2.1, 2.2

Supervising others: 4.2

Systems thinking: 1.1, 1.2, 1.3, 1.4, 2.1, 2.2

Time management: 4.1, 4.2

LEADER

Key competencies	Enabling competencies
PHYSICIANS ARE ABLE TO:	
1. **Contribute to the improvement of health care delivery in teams, organizations, and systems**	1.1 Apply the science of quality improvement to contribute to improving systems of patient care
	1.2 Contribute to a culture that promotes patient safety
	1.3 Analyze patient safety incidents to enhance systems of care
	1.4 Use health informatics to improve the quality of patient care and optimize patient safety
2. **Engage in the stewardship of health care resources**	2.1 Allocate health care resources for optimal patient care
	2.2 Apply evidence and management processes to achieve cost-appropriate care
3. **Demonstrate leadership in professional practice**	3.1 Demonstrate leadership skills to enhance health care
	3.2 Facilitate change in health care to enhance services and outcomes
4. **Manage career planning, finances, and health human resources in a practice**	4.1 Set priorities and manage time to integrate practice and personal life
	4.2 Manage a career and a practice
	4.3 Implement processes to ensure personal practice improvement

Health Advocate

DEFINITION

As Health Advocates, physicians contribute their expertise and influence as they work with communities or patient populations to improve health. They work with those they serve to determine and understand needs, speak on behalf of others when required, and support the mobilization of resources to effect change.

DESCRIPTION

Physicians are accountable to society and recognize their duty to contribute to efforts to improve the health and well-being of their patients, their communities, and the broader populations they serve.* Physicians possess medical knowledge and abilities that provide unique perspectives on health. Physicians also have privileged access to patients' accounts of their experience with illness and the health care system.

Improving health is not limited to mitigating illness or trauma, but also involves disease prevention, health promotion, and health protection. Improving health also includes promoting health equity, whereby individuals and populations reach their full health potential without being disadvantaged by, for example, race, ethnicity, religion, gender, sexual orientation, age, social class, economic status, or level of education.

Physicians leverage their position to support patients in navigating the health care system and to advocate with them to access appropriate resources in a timely manner. Physicians seek to improve the quality of both their clinical practice and associated organizations by addressing the health needs of the patients, communities, or populations they serve. Physicians promote healthy communities and populations by influencing the system (or by supporting others who influence the system), both within and outside of their work environments.

Advocacy requires action. Physicians contribute their knowledge of the determinants of health to positively influence the health of the patients, communities, or populations they serve. Physicians gather information and perceptions about issues, working with patients and their families[†] to develop an understanding of needs and potential mechanisms to address these needs. Physicians support patients, communities, or populations to call for change, and they speak on behalf of others when needed. Physicians increase awareness about important health issues at the patient, community, or population level. They support or lead the mobilization of resources (e.g. financial, material, or human resources) on small or large scales.

Physician advocacy occurs within complex systems and thus requires the development of partnerships with patients, their families and support networks, or community agencies and organizations to influence health determinants. Advocacy often requires engaging other health care professionals, community agencies, administrators, and policy-makers.

---

* In the CanMEDS 2015 Framework, a "community" is a group of people and/or patients connected to one's practice, and a "population" is a group of people and/or patients with a shared issue or characteristic.

† Throughout the CanMEDS 2015 Framework and Milestones Guide, references to the patient's family are intended to include all those who are personally significant to the patient and are concerned with his or her care, including, according to the patient's circumstances, family members, partners, caregivers, legal guardians, and substitute decision-makers.

KEY CONCEPTS

Adapting practice to respond to the needs of patients, communities, or populations served: 2.1, 2.2

Advocacy in partnership with patients, communities, and populations served: 1.1, 1.2, 2.1, 2.2, 2.3

Continuous quality improvement: 2.2, 2.3

Determinants of health, including psychological, biological, social, cultural, environmental, educational, and economic determinants, as well as health care system factors: 1.1, 1.3, 2.2

Disease prevention: 1.3, 2.1

Fiduciary duty: 1.1, 2.2, 2.3

Health equity: 2.2

Health promotion: 1.1, 1.2, 1.3, 2.1

Health protection: 1.3

Health system literacy: 1.1, 2.1

Mobilizing resources as needed: 1.1, 1.2, 1.3

Principles of health policy and its implications: 2.2

Potential for competing health interests of the individuals, communities, or populations served: 2.3

Responsible use of position and influence: 2.1, 2.3

Social accountability of physicians: 2.1, 2.3

Key competencies	Enabling competencies
PHYSICIANS ARE ABLE TO:	
1. **Respond to an individual patient's health needs by advocating with the patient within and beyond the clinical environment**	1.1 Work with patients to address determinants of health that affect them and their access to needed health services or resources
	1.2 Work with patients and their families to increase opportunities to adopt healthy behaviours
	1.3 Incorporate disease prevention, health promotion, and health surveillance into interactions with individual patients
2. **Respond to the needs of the communities or populations they serve by advocating with them for system-level change in a socially accountable manner**	2.1 Work with a community or population to identify the determinants of health that affect them
	2.2 Improve clinical practice by applying a process of continuous quality improvement to disease prevention, health promotion, and health surveillance activities
	2.3 Contribute to a process to improve health in the community or population they serve

Scholar

DEFINITION

As Scholars, physicians demonstrate a lifelong commitment to excellence in practice through continuous learning and by teaching others, evaluating evidence, and contributing to scholarship.

DESCRIPTION

Physicians acquire scholarly abilities to enhance practice and advance health care. Physicians pursue excellence by continually evaluating the processes and outcomes of their daily work, sharing and comparing their work with that of others, and actively seeking feedback in the interest of quality and patient safety. Using multiple ways of learning, they strive to meet the needs of individual patients and their families* and of the health care system.

Physicians strive to master their domains of expertise and to share their knowledge. As lifelong learners, they implement a planned approach to learning in order to improve in each CanMEDS Role. They recognize the need to continually learn and to model the practice of lifelong learning for others. As teachers they facilitate, individually and through teams, the education of students and physicians in training, colleagues, co-workers, the public, and others.

Physicians are able to identify pertinent evidence, evaluate it using specific criteria, and apply it in their practice and scholarly activities. Through their engagement in evidence-informed and shared decision-making, they recognize uncertainty in practice and formulate questions to address knowledge gaps. Using skills in navigating information resources, they identify evidence syntheses that are relevant to these questions and arrive at clinical decisions that are informed by evidence while taking patient values and preferences into account.

Finally, physicians' scholarly abilities allow them to contribute to the application, dissemination, translation, and creation of knowledge and practices applicable to health and health care.

KEY CONCEPTS

Lifelong learning
Collaborative learning: 1.3
Communities of practice: 1.3
Patient safety: 1.3
Performance assessment: 1.2
Personal learning plan: 1.1
Quality improvement: 1.1, 1.2, 1.3
Reflection on practice: 1.2
Seeking feedback: 1.2
Self-improvement: 1.1, 1.2, 1.3

Teacher
Faculty, rotation, and program evaluation: 2.5, 2.6
Formal and informal curricula: 2.1
Hidden curriculum: 2.1
Learner assessment: 2.5, 2.6
Learning outcomes: 2.4, 2.5, 2.6
Mentoring: 2.2, 2.5
Needs assessment: 2.4
Optimization of the learning environment: 2.2
Principles of assessment: 2.6
Providing feedback: 2.5, 2.6
Role-modelling: 2.1, 2.5
Supervision and graded responsibility: 2.3
Teaching and learning: 2.2, 2.4, 2.5

Evidence-informed decision-making
Effect size: 3.3, 3.4
Evidence-based medicine: 3.1, 3.2, 3.3, 3.4
Evidence synthesis: 3.2, 3.3
External validity: 3.3
Generalizability: 3.3
Information literacy: 3.2
Internal validity: 3.3
Knowledge gaps: 3.1
Knowledge translation: 3.3, 3.4
Quality-appraised evidence-alerting services: 3.2, 3.4
Recognizing bias in research: 3.3
Structured critical appraisal: 3.3
Uncertainty in practice: 3.1

Research
Conflict of interest: 4.2, 4.5
Confidentiality: 4.1, 4.2
Informed consent: 4.1
Research: 4.1, 4.2, 4.3, 4.5
Research ethics: 4.2
Research methods: 4.4
Scholarly inquiry: 4.1, 4.2, 4.4, 4.5
Scholarship: 4.1, 4.2
Scientific principles: 4.1

* Throughout the CanMEDS 2015 Framework and Milestones Guide, references to the patient's family are intended to include all those who are personally significant to the patient and are concerned with his or her care, including, according to the patient's circumstances, family members, partners, caregivers, legal guardians, and substitute decision-makers.

Key competencies	Enabling competencies
PHYSICIANS ARE ABLE TO:	
1. **Engage in the continuous enhancement of their professional activities through ongoing learning**	1.1 Develop, implement, monitor, and revise a personal learning plan to enhance professional practice 1.2 Identify opportunities for learning and improvement by regularly reflecting on and assessing their performance using various internal and external data sources 1.3 Engage in collaborative learning to continuously improve personal practice and contribute to collective improvements in practice
2. **Teach students, residents, the public, and other health care professionals**	2.1 Recognize the influence of role-modelling and the impact of the formal, informal, and hidden curriculum on learners 2.2 Promote a safe learning environment 2.3 Ensure patient safety is maintained when learners are involved 2.4 Plan and deliver a learning activity 2.5 Provide feedback to enhance learning and performance 2.6 Assess and evaluate learners, teachers, and programs in an educationally appropriate manner
3. **Integrate best available evidence into practice**	3.1 Recognize practice uncertainty and knowledge gaps in clinical and other professional encounters and generate focused questions that address them 3.2 Identify, select, and navigate pre-appraised resources 3.3 Critically evaluate the integrity, reliability, and applicability of health-related research and literature 3.4 Integrate evidence into decision-making in their practice
4. **Contribute to the creation and dissemination of knowledge and practices applicable to health**	4.1 Demonstrate an understanding of the scientific principles of research and scholarly inquiry and the role of research evidence in health care 4.2 Identify ethical principles for research and incorporate them into obtaining informed consent, considering potential harms and benefits, and considering vulnerable populations 4.3 Contribute to the work of a research program 4.4 Pose questions amenable to scholarly inquiry and select appropriate methods to address them 4.5 Summarize and communicate to professional and lay audiences, including patients and their families, the findings of relevant research and scholarly inquiry

PROFESSIONAL

Professional

DEFINITION

As Professionals, physicians are committed to the health and well-being of individual patients and society through ethical practice, high personal standards of behaviour, accountability to the profession and society, physician-led regulation, and maintenance of personal health.

DESCRIPTION*

Physicians serve an essential societal role as professionals dedicated to the health and care of others. Their work requires mastery of the art, science, and practice of medicine. A physician's professional identity is central to this Role. The Professional Role reflects contemporary society's expectations of physicians, which include clinical competence, a commitment to ongoing professional development, promotion of the public good, adherence to ethical standards, and values such as integrity, honesty, altruism, humility, respect for diversity, and transparency with respect to potential conflicts of interest. It is also recognized that, to provide optimal patient care, physicians must take responsibility for their own health and well-being and that of their colleagues. Professionalism is the basis of the implicit contract between society and the medical profession, granting the privilege of physician-led regulation with the understanding that physicians are accountable to those served, to society, to their profession, and to themselves.

KEY CONCEPTS

Professional identity: 1.1, 4.1, 4.2

Commitment to patients

Altruism: 1.1

Bioethical principles and theories: 1.3

Commitment to excellence in clinical practice and mastery of the discipline: 1.2

Compassion and caring: 1.1

Confidentiality and its limits: 1.1, 1.5

Disclosure of physician limitations that affect care: 1.1

Insight: 1.1, 1.3, 1.4, 2.1

Integrity and honesty: 1.1

Moral and ethical behaviour: 1.1, 1.3

Professional boundaries: 1.1

Respect for diversity: 1.1

Commitment to society

Commitment to the promotion of the public good in health care: 2.1, 2.2

Social accountability: 2.1, 2.2

Social contract in health care: 2.1, 2.2

Societal expectations of physicians and the profession: 2.1, 2.2

Commitment to the profession

Accountability to professional regulatory authorities: 3.1

Codes of ethics: 3.1

Commitment to patient safety and quality improvement: 2.1, 4.1

Commitment to professional standards: 3.1

Conflicts of interest (personal, financial, administrative, etc.): 1.4

Medico-legal frameworks governing practice: 3.1, 3.3

Responsibility to the profession, including obligations of peer assessment, mentorship, collegiality, and support: 3.2, 3.3, 4.3

---

* The Role description draws from Cruess SR, Johnston S, Cruess RL. "Profession": a working definition for medical educators. *Teach Learn Med.* 2004;16(1):74–6 and from Cruess SR, Cruess RL. Professionalism and medicine's social contract with society. *Virtual Mentor.* 2004;6(4).

Commitment to self

Applied capacity for self-regulation, including the assessment and monitoring of one's thoughts, behaviours, emotions, and attention for optimal performance and well-being: 4.1

Career development and career transitions: 4.1, 4.2

Commitment to disclosure of harmful patient safety incidents, including those resulting from medical error, and their impact: 4.2, 4.3

Mindful and reflective approach to practice: 4.2

Resilience for sustainable practice: 4.2

Responsibility to self, including personal care, in order to serve others: 4.1

Key competencies	Enabling competencies
PHYSICIANS ARE ABLE TO:	
1. **Demonstrate a commitment to patients by applying best practices and adhering to high ethical standards**	1.1 Exhibit appropriate professional behaviours and relationships in all aspects of practice, demonstrating honesty, integrity, humility, commitment, compassion, respect, altruism, respect for diversity, and maintenance of confidentiality
	1.2 Demonstrate a commitment to excellence in all aspects of practice
	1.3 Recognize and respond to ethical issues encountered in practice
	1.4 Recognize and manage conflicts of interest
	1.5 Exhibit professional behaviours in the use of technology-enabled communication
2. **Demonstrate a commitment to society by recognizing and responding to societal expectations in health care**	2.1 Demonstrate accountability to patients, society, and the profession by responding to societal expectations of physicians
	2.2 Demonstrate a commitment to patient safety and quality improvement
3. **Demonstrate a commitment to the profession by adhering to standards and participating in physician-led regulation**	3.1 Fulfill and adhere to the professional and ethical codes, standards of practice, and laws governing practice
	3.2 Recognize and respond to unprofessional and unethical behaviours in physicians and other colleagues in the health care professions
	3.3 Participate in peer assessment and standard-setting
4. **Demonstrate a commitment to physician health and well-being to foster optimal patient care**	4.1 Exhibit self-awareness and manage influences on personal well-being and professional performance
	4.2 Manage personal and professional demands for a sustainable practice throughout the physician life cycle
	4.3 Promote a culture that recognizes, supports, and responds effectively to colleagues in need

A taxonomy of physician competencies

Competence refers to the abilities needed to practice effectively within a defined scope and context. The following taxonomy is designed to explain the structure of the CanMEDS Physician Competency Framework and its application to a program. While each physician has a unique set of abilities, in everyday practice these competencies are integrated into a seamless whole and reflect the daily activities of the physician.

CanMEDS Roles. The CanMEDS Framework is organized into seven thematic groups of competencies, which are expressed as physician Roles. While the Roles are clearly synergistic and interrelated, they are also unique. In this way, a Role can be described as a *meta-competency.*

Key competencies. Within each CanMEDS Role, there are a defined number of essential abilities known as key competencies. The key competencies refer to the knowledge, skills, and attitudes of a physician and are described as global educational statements.

Enabling competencies. The term "enabling competencies" refers to the essential components of a key competency. Several enabling competencies in concert describe in greater detail the components of a key competency.

CanMEDS Milestones. CanMEDS Milestones illustrate the expected progression of competence from *novice to mastery* associated with each enabling competency. CanMEDS Milestones assist learners, curriculum designers, and clinical teachers to determine where a person is situated in their progress towards competence. These Milestones are organized against the Competence Continuum (see Milestones section).

DISCIPLINE-SPECIFIC COMPETENCIES

Each Specialty Committee of the Royal College applies a discipline-specific lens to the CanMEDS Roles, key and enabling competencies, and milestones to reflect its unique practice. The Specialty Committee expresses the competencies as educational statements that make up each discipline's training standards.

Royal College Entrustable Professional Activities (RCEPAs). Royal College Entrustable Professional Activities refer to the tasks in a professional setting that may be delegated to a physician once competence in the task has been demonstrated. RCEPAs incorporate multiple CanMEDS Milestones from various CanMEDS Roles. RCEPAs allow for authentic, work-based assessment that is targeted at the daily tasks of physicians.

PROGRAM OBJECTIVES

Program objectives refer to discipline-specific statements describing the specific educational goals of a curriculum derived from the CanMEDS competencies, such as those used for a residency or continuing professional development program.

Key contributors

EXPERT WORKING GROUPS

With input from key partners, the Royal College assembled 11 Expert Working Groups (EWGs) to examine the seven core CanMEDS domains; of these groups, four focused on distinct aspects of the Scholar domain and two focused on aspects of the Professional domain. All of the groups were advised by two additional EWGs on integrating new content related to patient safety and quality improvement and to eHealth respectively across the seven CanMEDS Roles.

Each EWG was composed of medical educators and practising physicians from a range of specialties (i.e., representatives from the College of Family Physicians of Canada, Collège des médecins du Québec and Royal College) and provinces. Students and trainees were included wherever possible. The EWGs were tasked with:

- reviewing the CanMEDS 2005 Framework to identify concepts potentially requiring clarification or modification, as well as any gaps or redundancies in the competencies;

- incorporating new themes such as patient safety, quality improvement and eHealth into the framework;

- developing draft milestones for each CanMEDS Role;

- ensuring that the framework is practical and useful for education across the continuum; and

- acting on feedback from consultations and integrating relevant content into the revised CanMEDS Framework.

MEDICAL EXPERT

Chair
Dr. Farhan Bhanji, McGill University

Core members
Dr. Kathy Lawrence, College of Family Physicians of Canada
Dr. Mark Goldszmidt, University of Western Ontario
Dr. Mark Walton, McMaster University
Dr. Kenneth Harris, Royal College of Physicians and Surgeons of Canada
Dr. David Creery, University of Ottawa
Dr. Jonathan Sherbino, McMaster University

Dr. Louis-George Ste-Marie, Université de Montréal
Dr. Antonia Stang, University of Calgary

Advisory
Dr. Ivy F Oandasan, College of Family Physicians of Canada

Project coordinator
Marvel Sampson

COMMUNICATOR

Chair
Dr. Alan Neville, McMaster University

Core members
Dr. Wayne Weston, University of Western Ontario
Dr. Dawn Martin, University of Toronto
Dr. Louise Samson, Collège des médecins du Québec
Dr. Perle Feldman, College of Family Physicians of Canada
Dr. Gordon Wallace, Canadian Medical Protective Association
Dr. Olivier Jamoulle, Université de Montréal
Dr. José François, University of Manitoba
Dr. Marie-Thérèse Lussier, Université de Montréal
Dr. Sue Dojeiji, University of Ottawa

Advisory
Dr. Judy Brown, College of Family Physicians of Canada
Dr. Erin Keely, University of Ottawa
Dr. Suzanne Kurtz, University of Calgary (Emerita)
Ms. Abigail Hain, Canadian Patient Safety Institute

Project coordinators
Cynthia Abbott
Ginette Bourgeois

COLLABORATOR

Chair
Dr. Denyse Richardson, University of Toronto

Core members
Dr. Lisa Calder, University of Ottawa
Dr. Heather Dean, University of Manitoba
Dr. Susan Glover Takahashi, University of Toronto
Dr. Paule Lebel, Université de Montréal

KEY CONTRIBUTORS

Dr. Jerry Maniate, University of Toronto
Dr. Dawn Martin, University of Toronto
Dr. Louise Nasmith, College of Family Physicians of Canada
Dr. Christie Newton, College of Family Physicians of Canada
Dr. Yvonne Steinert, McGill University

Advisory
Dr. Amir Ginzburg, University of Toronto
Dr. Ivy F Oandasan, College of Family Physicians of Canada
Dr. Sharon Switzer-McIntyre, University of Toronto

Project coordinator
Wendy Jemmett

LEADER (was Manager)

Chairs
Dr. Deepak Dath, McMaster University
Dr. Ming-Ka Chan, University of Manitoba

Core members
Dr. Geoffrey Anderson, University of Toronto
Dr. Andrew Burke, University of Western Ontario
Dr. Saleem Razack, McGill University
Dr. Susan Lieff, University of Toronto
Dr. Geneviève Moineau, Association of Faculties of Medicine of Canada
Dr. Aaron Chiu, University of Manitoba
Dr. Philip Ellison, College of Family Physicians of Canada

Advisory
Dr. David Snadden, University of British Columbia
Mr. Hugh MacLeod, Canadian Patient Safety Institute
Dr. Sherissa Microys, University of Ottawa
Dre Marie-Josée Bédard, Université of Montréal
Dr. Joshua Tepper, Health Quality Ontario
Dr. Louis-André Lacasse, Université de Montréal
Dr. Hema Patel, McGill University

Project coordinators
Cynthia Abbott
Mélanie Agnew
Ginette Bourgeois

HEALTH ADVOCATE

Chair
Dr. Jonathan Sherbino, McMaster University

Core members
Dr. Deirdre Bonnycastle, University of Saskatchewan
Dr. Brigitte Côté, Université de Montréal
Dr. Leslie Flynn, Queen's University
Dr. Andrea Hunter, McMaster University
Dr. Daniel Ince-Cushman, College of Family Physicians of Canada
Dr. Jill Konkin, University of Alberta
Dr. Ivy F Oandasan, College of Family Physicians of Canada
Dr. Glenn Regehr, University of British Columbia
Dr. Denyse Richardson, University of Toronto
Dr. Jean Zigby, College of Family Physicians of Canada

Advisory
Dr. Marcia Clark, University of Calgary
Dr. Sherissa Microys, University of Ottawa

Project coordinator
Marvel Sampson

SCHOLAR

Chairs
Dr. Denyse Richardson, University of Toronto
Dr. Anna Oswald, University of Alberta

Scholar – Lifelong Learning
Chair
Dr. Denyse Richardson, University of Toronto

Core members
Dr. Nathalie Caire Fon, Université de Montréal
Dr. Craig Campbell, Royal College of Physicians and Surgeons of Canada
Dr. Ian Goldstine, College of Family Physicians of Canada
Ms. Jennifer Gordon, Royal College of Physicians and Surgeons of Canada
Dr. Jocelyn Lockyer, University of Calgary
Dr. Karen Mann, Dalhousie University
Dr. John Parboosingh, University of Calgary
Dr. Mithu Sen, University of Western Ontario
Dr. Ivan Silver, University of Toronto

Advisory
Dr. Robert Bluman, University of British Columbia
Dr. Dave Davis, Association of American Medical Colleges
Dr. François Goulet, Collège des médecins du Québec
Dr. Brenna Lynn, University of British Columbia
Dr. Jamie Meuser, College of Family Physicians of Canada
Dr. Brian M Wong, University of Toronto

Project coordinator
Wendy Jemmett

Scholar – Teacher
Chairs
Dr. Anna Oswald, University of Alberta
Dr. Ming-Ka Chan, University of Manitoba

Core members
Dr. Karen Mann, Dalhousie University
Dr. Wayne Weston, University of Western Ontario
Dr. Elisa Ruano Cea, McGill University
Dr. Constance LeBlanc, Dalhousie University
Dr. Farhan Bhanji, McGill University
Dr. James Goertzen, College of Family Physicians of Canada
Dr. Jennifer Walton, University of Alberta
Dr. Marcia Clark, University of Calgary
Dr. Brian M Wong, University of Toronto

Advisory
Dr. Nick Busing, Future of Medical Education in Canada Postgraduate
Dr. Sal Spadafora, University of Toronto
Dr. Allyn Walsh, College of Family Physicians of Canada
Dr. Chris Watling, University of Western Ontario

Project coordinator
Ginette Bourgeois
Marvel Sampson

Scholar – Critical Appraisal
Chair
Dr. Eddy S Lang, University of Calgary

Core members
Dr. Martin Dawes, University of British Columbia
Dr. Roland Grad, McGill University
Dr. Brian Haynes, McMaster University
Dr. Jim Henderson, McGill University

Ms. Lorie Kloda, McGill University
Ms. Susan Powelson, University of Calgary

Advisory
Dr. Lisa Calder, University of Ottawa
Dr. Julien Poitras, Université Laval
Dr. Kent Stobart, University of Alberta

Project coordinators
Ginette Bourgeois
Cynthia MacLachlan
Shelley Murdock

Scholar – Research
Chair
Dr. Bart J Harvey, University of Toronto

Core members
Dr. Stacy Ackroyd-Stolarz, Dalhousie University
Dr. Tanya Horsley, Royal College of Physicians and Surgeons of Canada
Dr. Vivian R Ramsden, College of Family Physicians of Canada
Dr. David Streiner, University of Toronto

Project coordinator
Wendy Jemmett

PROFESSIONAL

Chairs
Dr. Linda Snell, McGill University
Dr. Leslie Flynn, Queen's University

Professionalism
Chair
Dr. Linda Snell, McGill University

Core members
Dr. Leslie Flynn, Queen's University
Dr. Merril Pauls, College of Family Physicians of Canada
Dr. Ramona Kearney, University of Alberta
Dr. Andrew Warren, Dalhousie University
Dr. Robert Sternszus, McGill University
Dr. Richard Cruess, McGill University
Dr. Sylvia Cruess, McGill University
Dr. Maggy Dupré, Collège des médecins du Québec
Dr. Rose Hatala, Collège des médecins du Québec

KEY CONTRIBUTORS

Advisory
Dr. Shiphra Ginsburg, University or Toronto
Dr. Sharon Johnston, University of Ottawa
Dr. Yvette Lajeunesse, Université de Montreal

Project coordinator
Tammy Hesson

Physician Health
Chair
Dr. Leslie Flynn, Queen's University

Core members
Dr. Linda Snell, McGill University
Dr. Meri Bukowskyj, Canadian Medical Protective Association
Dr. Susan Edwards, College of Family Physicians of Canada
Dr. Jordan Cohen, University of Calgary
Dr. Anita Chakravarti, University of Saskatchewan
Dr. Leslie Nickell, University of Toronto
Dr. Janet Wright, College of Physicians and Surgeons of Alberta

Advisory
Dr. Jonathan DellaVedova, McGill University (resident)
Dr. Eva Knell, College of Family Physicians of Canada
Dr. Derek Puddester, Canadian Medical Association
Dr. Andrew Warren, Dalhousie University

Project coordinator
Tammy Hesson

PATIENT SAFETY AND QUALITY IMPROVEMENT
Chair
Dr. Brian M Wong, University of Toronto

Core members
Dr. Stacy Ackroyd-Stolarz, Dalhousie University
Dr. Meri Bukowskyj, Canadian Medical Protective Association
Dr. Lisa Calder, University of Ottawa
Dr. Amir Ginzberg, University of Toronto
Dr. Sherissa Microys, University of Ottawa
Dr. Antonia Stang, University of Calgary
Dr. Gordon Wallace, Canadian Medical Protective Association

Advisory
Dr. Philip Ellison, University of Toronto
Dr. Ward Flemons, University of Calgary
Ms. Abigail Hain, Canadian Patient Safety Institute
Dr. Karen Hall Barber, Queen's University
Dr. Amy Nakajima, University of Ottawa
Dr. Kaveh Shojana, University of Toronto
Dr. Roger Wong, University of British Columbia

Project coordinator
Tammy Hesson

eHEALTH
Chair
Dr. Kendall Ho, University of British Columbia

Core members
Dr. Rachel Ellaway, Northern Ontario School of Medicine
Dr. Judith Littleford, University of Manitoba
Dr. Robert Hayward, University of Alberta
Dr. Katrina Hurley, Dalhousie University

Project coordinator
Marvel Sampson

CANMEDS 2015 NATIONAL ADVISORY COMMITTEE

The CanMEDS 2015 National Advisory Committee provided strategic direction and input on the overall CanMEDS 2015 project and included representatives from a range of key stakeholders and partner organizations.

Chairs
Dr. Jason R Frank, Royal College of Physicians and Surgeons of Canada
Dr. Ivy F Oandasan, College of Family Physicians of Canada

Members
Ms. Cynthia Abbott, Royal College of Physicians and Surgeons of Canada
Dr. Adelle Atkinson, University of Toronto
Dr. Glen Bandiera, University of Toronto
Dr. Andrée Boucher, Université de Montréal

Dr. Ian Bowmer, Medical Council of Canada

Dr. Ian Brasg, Canadian Federation of Medical Students

Dr. Ford Bursey, Memorial University

Dr. Nick Busing, Future of Medical Education in Canada Postgraduate

Dr. François Caron, Fédération des médecins résidents du Québec

Dr. Charles Faubert, Fédération des médecins résidents du Québec

Dr. Katharine Gillis, University of Ottawa

Dr. Lisa Graves, Northern Ontario School of Medicine, Undergraduate Dean

Dr. Kenneth Harris, Royal College of Physicians and Surgeons of Canada

Dr. Kevin Imrie, Royal College of Physicians and Surgeons of Canada

Dr. Fleur-Ange Lefebvre, Federation of Medical Regulatory Authorities of Canada

Dr. Anne Marie MacLellan, Collège des médecins du Québec

Mr. Hugh MacLeod, Canadian Patient Safety Institute

Dr. Ashley Miller, Resident Doctors of Canada

Dr. Geneviève Moineau, Association of Faculties of Medicine of Canada

Dr. Julien Poitras, Université Laval, Postgraduate Dean

Dr. Charmaine Roye, Canadian Medical Association

Dr. Kam Rungta, Royal College of Physicians and Surgeons of Canada

Dr. Asoka Samarasena, Memorial University, Postgraduate Dean

Dr. Linda Snell, Royal College of Physicians and Surgeons of Canada

Dr. Kent Stobart, University of Alberta, Undergraduate Dean

Dr. Gary Tithecott, University of Western Ontario, Undergraduate Dean

Dr. Gordon Wallace, Canadian Medical Protective Association

Dr. Parveen Wasi, McMaster University

Dr. James Wilson, Royal College Education Committee

Dr. Roger Wong, University of British Columbia, Postgraduate Dean

Project coordinator
Tammy Hesson

CANMEDS 2015 INTERNATIONAL ADVISORY COMMITTEE

The CanMEDS 2015 International Advisory Committee was convened to provide input on the overall CanMEDS 2015 project from a global perspective, with a view to the potential impact of the revised framework in other countries and jurisdictions. Members included representatives from a range of international stakeholders and partner organizations.

Chairs

Dr. Jason R Frank, Royal College of Physicians and Surgeons of Canada, Canada

Dr. Linda Snell, Royal College of Physicians and Surgeons of Canada, Canada

Members

Dr. Ducksun Ahn, Korea

Dr. Esam Al Banyan, Saudi Arabia

Dr. Andleeb Arshad, Kuwait

Dr. Sally Davies, United Kingdom

Dr. Jean-François Denef, Belgium

Dr. Peter Dieckmann, Denmark

Dr. Richard Doherty, Australia

Dr. Robert Englander, United States of America

Dr. Jaime Godoy, Chili

Dr. Peter Harris, Australia

Dr. Jennie Kendrick, Australia

Dr. Scott Lang, Australia/Canada

Dr. Mary Lawson, Australia

Dr. Haicho Li, China

Dr. Tindal Magnus, Australia

Dr. Doris Ostergaard, Denmark

Dr. Ingrid Philibert, United States of America

Dr. Peter Raubenheimer, South Africa

Dr. Fedde Scheele, Netherlands

Dr. Stefanus Snyman, South Africa

Dr. Marie-Louise Stokes, Australia

Dr. Tim Swanwick, England

Dr. Olle ten Cate, Netherlands

Mr. Patrick van Gele, Switzerland

Dr. Simon Williams, Australia

Project coordinator
Marvel Sampson

KEY CONTRIBUTORS

THE ROYAL COLLEGE INTEGRATION COMMITTEE

A small team of clinician educators from across Canada was commissioned to synthesize the contributions to the CanMEDS 2015 project into a coherent version of the 2015 Framework and the complementary Milestones Guide. These contributions included EWG reports, directions from the National and International Advisory Committees, survey and focus group results, summaries of town hall discussions, informal feedback and reports from sister institutions worldwide.

Chairs
Dr. Jason R Frank, Royal College of Physicians and Surgeons of Canada
Dr. Linda Snell, McGill University

Members
Ms. Cynthia Abbott, Royal College of Physicians and Surgeons of Canada
Dr. Craig Campbell, Royal College of Physicians and Surgeons of Canada
Dr. Kenneth Harris, Royal College of Physicians and Surgeons of Canada
Dr. Farhan Bhanji, McGill University
Dr. Andrée Boucher, Université de Montréal
Dr. Ming-Ka Chan, University of Manitoba
Dr. Lara Cooke, University of Calgary
Dr. Deepak Dath, McMaster University
Dr. Sue Dojeiji, University of Ottawa
Dr. Leslie Flynn, Queen's University
Ms. Danielle Frechette, Royal College of Physicians and Surgeons of Canada
Ms. Jennifer Gordon, Royal College of Physicians and Surgeons of Canada
Dr. Jolanta Karpinski, Royal College of Physicians and Surgeons of Canada
Dr. Viren Naik, University of Ottawa
Dr. Anna Oswald, University of Alberta
Dr. Denyse Richardson, University of Toronto
Dr. Jonathan Sherbino, McMaster University
Dr. Elaine Van Melle, Queen's University

Project coordinator
Tammy Hesson

ROYAL COLLEGE FRENCH ADVISORY COMMITTEE

The Royal College French Advisory Committee members closely examined the French versions of the CanMEDS 2015 Physician Competency Framework and the CanMEDS 2015 Milestones. Through their careful review of the documents, the Committee members made strategic changes to reflect the current discourse in medical education and practice.

Chair
Dr. Andrée Boucher, Université de Montréal

Members
Dr. Paul Belliveau, Queen's University
Dr. José François, University of Manitoba
Ms. Lucie Hamelin, College of Family Physicians of Canada
Dr. Jean Latreille, Université de Sherbrooke
Dr. Jean-François Lemay, University of Calgary
Dr. Julien Poitras, Université Laval
Dr. Serge Quérin, Université de Montréal
Dr. Louise Samson, Collège des médecins du Québec
Dr. Louis-George Ste-Marie, Université de Montréal

Project coordinator
Ginette Bourgeois

Translation support
Martin Côté
Nathalie Upton

CANMEDS 2015 PROJECT SECRETARIAT

Project Advisor
Cynthia Abbott

Project Team
Mélanie Agnew
Ginette Bourgeois
Caroline Clouston
Lana Dixon
Tammy Hesson
Wendy Jemmett
Cynthia MacLachlan
Sarah Matthews
Megan McComb
Shelley Murdock
Marvel Sampson
Kate Slean

References

1   Busing N, MacLellan A-M, Oandasan I, Harris K. *A Collective Vision for Postgraduate Medical Education in Canada*. Ottawa: The Future of Medical Education in Canada, FMEC PG Project Report. Collège des médecins du Québec, The College of Family Physicians of Canada, Royal College of Physicians and Surgeons of Canada; 2012. Available from: https://www.afmc.ca/medical-education/future-medical-education-canada-fmec

2   Quoted in Snyder L. *The Philosophical Breakfast Club*. New York: Random House; 2011.

3   Neufeld VR, Maudsley RF, Pickering RJ, Turnbull JM, Weston WW, Brown MG, Simpson JC. Educating future physicians for Ontario. *Acad Med*. 1998;73(11):1133–48.

4   Maudsley RF, Wilson DR, Neufeld VR, Hennen BK, DeVillaer MR, Wakefield J, MacFadyen J, Turnbull JM, Weston WW, Brown MG, Frank JR, Richardson D. Educating future physicians for Ontario: phase II. *Acad Med*. 2000;75(2):113–26.

5   Frank, JR. The CanMEDS project: The Royal College of Physicians and Surgeons of Canada moves medical education into the 21st century. In: Dinsdale HB, Hurteau G, editors. *The Royal College of Physicians and Surgeons of Canada: the evolution of specialty medicine, 1979–2004*. Ottawa: Royal College of Physicians and Surgeons of Canada; 2005. (p.187–98)

6   Frank JR, editor. *The CanMEDS 2005 Physician Competency Framework*. Better standards. Better physicians. Better care. Ottawa: Royal College of Physicians and Surgeons of Canada; 2005.

7   royalcollege.ca/cbd

8   Frank JR, Snell L, ten Cate O, Holmboe ES, Carraccio C, Swing SR, Harris P, Glasgow NJ, Campbell C, Dath D, Harden RM, Iobst W, Long DM, Mungroo R, Richardson DL, Sherbino J, Silver I, Taber S, Talbot M, Harris KA. Competency-based medical education: theory to practice. *Med Teach*. 2010;32(8):638–45.

9   www.royalcollege.ca/canmeds2015-ewg-report-1

10 Abbott C, Bourgeois G, Frank JR, MacLachlan C, Ronson A, and Van Melle E. *What we heard: Sharing the results of the CanMEDS 2015 Series I and II consultations*. Ottawa: Royal College of Physicians and Surgeons of Canada; 2014.

11 Frank JR, Snell L, Sherbino J, Boucher A, rédacteurs. *Référentiel de compétences CanMEDS 2015 pour les médecins*. Ottawa: Collège royal des médecins et chirurgiens du Canada; 2015.

12 Sherbino J, Frank JR, Flynn L, Snell L. "Intrinsic Roles" rather than "armour", renaming the "non-medical expert roles" of the CanMEDS framework to match their intent. *Adv in Health Sci Educ. Theory Prac*. 2011;16(5):695–7.

13 Van Melle E. *New and emerging concepts as related to the CanMEDS Roles*. Ottawa: Royal College of Physicians and Surgeons of Canada; 2013.

14 Aggarwal R, Darzi A. Technical-skills training in the 21st century. *N Engl J Med* 2006;355(25):2695–6.

NOTES